What's Below Your Tummy-Tum?

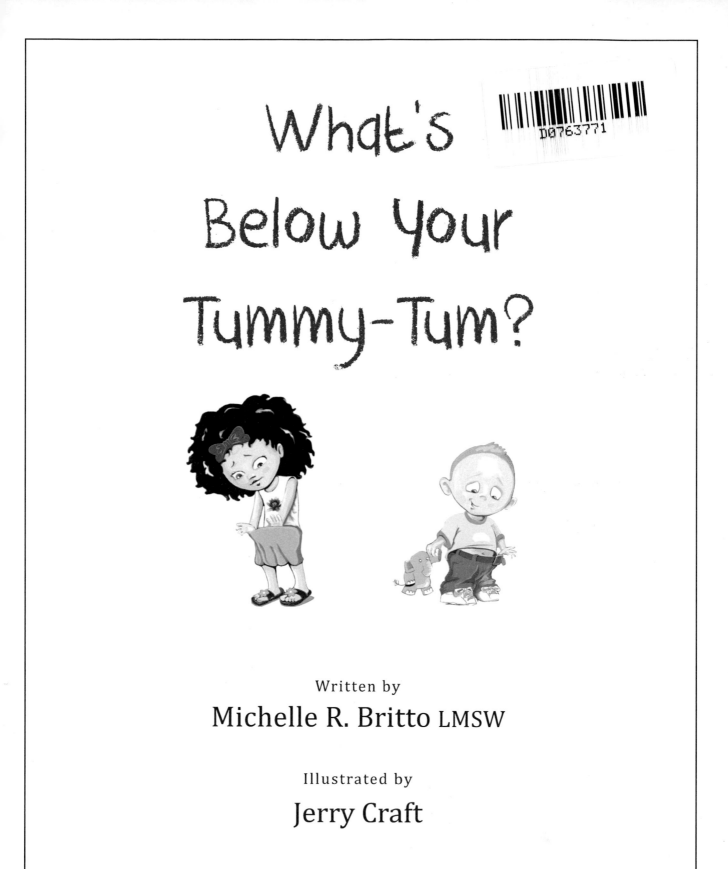

Written by

Michelle R. Britto LMSW

Illustrated by

Jerry Craft

InLightenMe Books • New York

What's Below Your Tummy-Tum?
Written by Michelle R. Britto
Illustrated by Jerry Craft
Book Design by Danni Ai courtesy of DACCo Multimedia, Inc
Edited by Randall Horton

Visit us on the web at http://www.inlightenmebooks.com

Follow @inlightenmebook on Twitter

Summary: Meet *Lotus* and *Nesh,* two children who, with the help of their guides *Li'l Lotus* and *Li'l Neshi,* learn about their private areas and how to keep them safe. This book was written by a social worker to teach and empower kids to protect themselves from people and situations that may cause them harm.

Soft Cover ISBN-13: 978-0-9884218-1-3
Soft Cover ISBN-10: 098842181X
Hard Cover ISBN-13: 978-0-9884218-2-0
Hard Cover ISBN-10: 0988421828

Library of Congress Control Number: 2013901009

First Edition
Printed in the United States

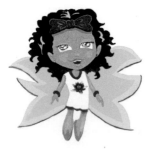

Published by InLightenMe Books

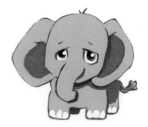

THANK YOU!

This book is dedicated to my daughter, Ariah-Lan, whose energy birthed this book to life. To Ava Jade, Aniya and Nancy. Ellijah, my first love; Jahsiah, never be afraid; Ryan and Jose who turned pain into triumph. To the givers of MY Breath: my parents Paulette and Michael Britto; my grandmothers Anna Broushet and Felicita Ramos; Eric and George Mussig, you nurtured me. To Myrtle Davis, my guardian angel on Earth who hears silent cries. And last but not least, the children and adults all over the world who will be empowered to breathe from this book.

Special thanks to Rev. Dr. Michael Bernard Beckwith for seeing my light and being authentically beautiful; his wife Rickie BB for her empowering words; Marta Lucia Garcia for reminding me of the importance of Energy; Gloria Rodriguez, my intuitive realist with a heart; Wayne Headley and for believing in me; Gina Heard for keeping it compassionate and real and giving voice to so many; Patrick Oliver for his knowledge and support and for introducing me to my phenomenal illustrator Jerry Craft. To Erin Neill Williams, Tracette Hillman and Glen Williams Jr. with gratitude; And most important, ALL of my family and friends who supported me through birthing this dream to promote safety in children through empowerment.

A Message from the Author

This book was written as a labor of love. As a social worker, I see so many children who are the victims of events that will change their little lives forever. It is my hope, that together, we can prepare them, and teach them ahead of time, in order to preserve their innocence and have them live a happy and healthy childhood.

You'll meet **Lotus** and **Nesh** and their guides **Li'l Lotus** and **Li'l Neshi**. Lotus is a little girl named after a pretty flower that grows out of murky water, like no other, and develops a strong stem that can withstand almost anything. It opens and closes based on what it needs for survival. The Lotus flower has always been symbolic throughout many aspects of the Chinese culture.

Nesh is her friend whose name is derived from Ganesh, which symbolizes the removal of obstacles in many parts of the East Indian culture. I named him Nesh to represent the removal of unnecessary obstacles by empowering our children.

You'll notice before you turn each page there are instructions for the reader and child to take a moment to breathe. This is important because breathing resets and grounds the body. The power of taking a breath helps to reaffirm what you've learned on each page. This exercise will empower children by teaching them to self-regulate mind, body and spirit.

Finally, as you read along, make sure to explain to your child that this book is to teach them to protect their privacy. But as a mom, dad or guardian, there will be times when you may have to see their bodies; bath time, doctor visits, checking for boo-boos, etc ...

Children are born into a world of so many things, but if we give a strong foundation and educate them, they will blossom and have the inner wisdom to protect themselves, opening and closing when necessary.

Thank you,

Michelle R. Britto

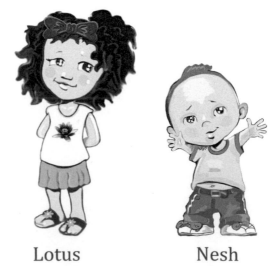

Lotus   Nesh

What's below your *Tummy-Tum*?
What's below yours and mine?
What's below his and hers?
What could it be?
Is it for everyone to **see**?
No way!
That should *NEVER* **be.**

Breathe in nice and deep, no matter what your age, then let it out slowly before you turn the page.

Do you know where your *Tummy-Tum* is?
Touch your *Tummy-Tum,* please.
Now, right below it is your very private **part**,
and learning to keep this safe
is where we will **start**.

PRIVATE means that it's special,
like a work of **art**,
so it should not be seen
or touched
by anyone but you,
Dear **Heart**.

These are not the body parts
you use when you are at **play**.
They *are* the ones you need
when you use the potty
each **day**.

Breathe in and breathe out nice and slow, breathe in really deeply, then let it go.

If you're a girl,
your private body part
is called a **VAGINA**.
It almost sounds
like the place called *China*.

What do *you* call it?

If you're a boy,
then your part is not the **same**.
It's even called by another **name**.
It almost sounds
like the word *peanuts*,
but it's **not**.
If you're a boy,
then a *PENIS*
is what you've **got**.

What do *you*
call it?

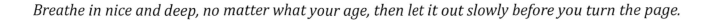

Breathe in nice and deep, no matter what your age, then let it out slowly before you turn the page.

They should really stay private inside your **underwear**. Whether you're a boy or a girl you should learn to be **aware**.

Your body, your mind and your little **heart**, these are the things you must learn to **protect** from the very **start**.

PRIVATE

Now PRIVATE is a word
that we already **know**.
It means only for you,
and it's not for **show**.
So when you put on clothes
or go to the **potty**,
do not let ANYONE
see your little **body**.

Breathe in and breathe out nice and slow, breathe in really deeply, then let it go.

The list of private parts
is not **complete**,
without the one you use
to sit on a **seat**.
It's called your butt,
or your booty,
or some call it a **rump**.
It's in the back of your pants
looking like two little **humps**.

What do *you* call it?

Now think about when you need private **time**.
Or a space where you say,
"this is **mine**!"
The bathroom? Your bedroom?
That's good to **know**.
I can feel that your power
is really starting to **grow**.

Breathe in nice and deep, no matter what your age, then let it out slowly before you turn the page.

Now this is **key**,
so listen closely to **me**.
With your eyes, you see ...

With your ears,
you hear ...

With your mouth,
you **eat** ...

But your mouth also
gives other treats ...

... like KISSES,
which can be really **sweet**.
But they do not belong
on everyone's **cheek**.

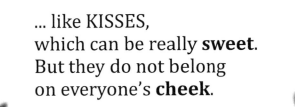

Kisses are given only when you say **so**.
Just remember, you have the power
to always say "**NO!**"

Breathe in and breathe out nice and slow, breathe in really deeply, then let it go.

Now say it **LOUD**,
and say it **PROUD!**
"I am the power
so remember my **name** ...

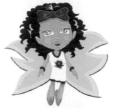

I do **NOT** play
the-below-
my-Tummy-Tum-
touching-game."

Playing games can be so much **fun**,
but when BAD touching starts,
the game is **done**!
Touching is not for **everyone**.
Yell for help and try to **run**!

Breathe in nice and deep, no matter what your age, then let it out slowly before you turn the page.

STOP touching me
when I **say**,
"No thank you!
No more **play**!"
Say it loud
to make them go **away**.
This is a place
you should not **stay**!

What's on *MY* body belongs to **me**.
It's only for *ME* to **see**.
What's on *YOUR* body is just for **you**,
it's not for *ME* to touch or **view**

Now you're rooted.
That means you're really strong.
Strong is how you belong.

Breathe in and breathe out nice and slow, breathe in really deeply, then let it go.

"I AM THE POWER,"
is what you **say**,
if someone won't
leave you alone,
or won't go **away**.
Tell them: "Touching
games are not for **me**,
I'm just a kid
so let me **be**!"

Now the word SAFE means you feel happy and **free**.
Around *safe people* is where you want to **be**.
Safe people, you do not send **away**.
They help to protect you night and **day**.

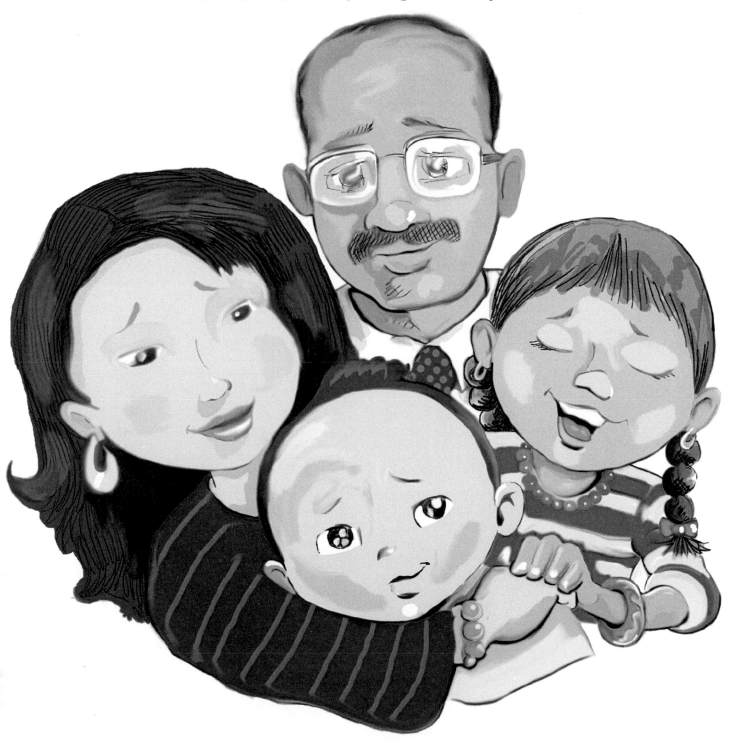

Breathe in nice and deep, no matter what your age, then let it out slowly before you turn the page.

Keep yourself safe, so you never have to **fear**.
No one can hurt you, when you make yourself **clear**.
Think about the safe people who you keep **near**,
these are the people who really hold you **dear**.

Who are the safe *Women* or *Girls* in your life? They *could be* moms, sisters, friends, aunts, teachers, grandmothers ... Make a list below, then have an adult make their list.

Child's list:

_____

_____

_____

_____

_____

_____

Adult's list:

_____

_____

_____

_____

_____

_____

List the names you both agree on:

_____

_____

_____

_____

Bath time, playing in the grass time,
and changing your little pants time,
are all for the safe people you **know**.
When you're around them you can

GROW ... **GROW... GROW!**

Who are the safe *Men* or *Boys*
in your life? They *could be* dads,
brothers, friends, uncles, teachers,
grandfathers ... Make a list below,
then have an adult make their list.

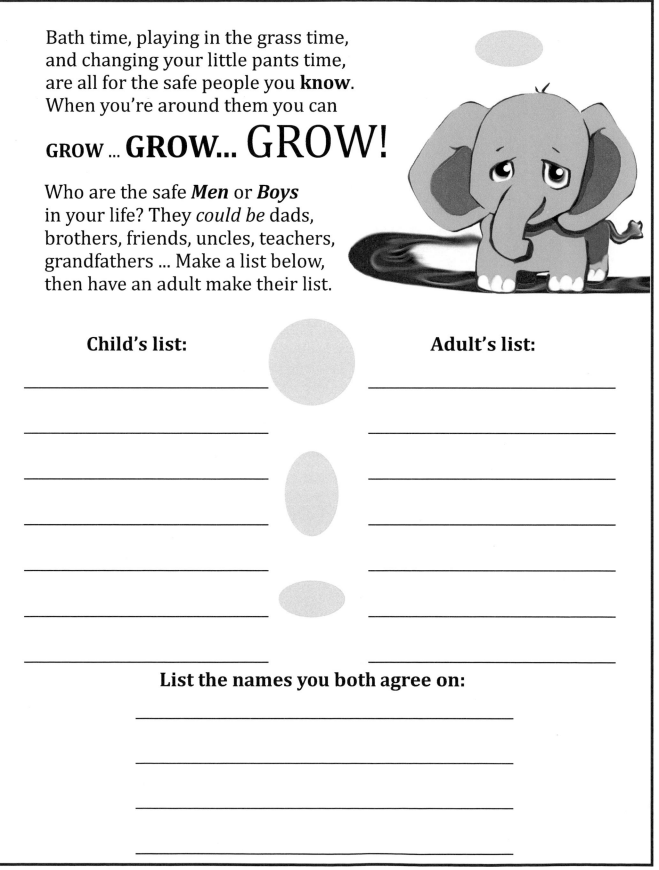

Child's list: **Adult's list:**

_____   _____

_____   _____

_____   _____

_____   _____

_____   _____

List the names you both agree on:

_____

_____

_____

_____

Breathe in and breathe out nice and slow, breathe in really deeply, then let it go.

Here is another important word to know: SECRETS!
Surprises are good things that make you feel **glad**,
but sometimes secrets will make you feel **sad**.
A secret is very different from a **surprise**,
and you should never be forced to
keep them, if they are **lies**.

Secrets can be fun between you and your **friends**,
but when secrets are bad, that's when the fun **ends**.
Don't ever keep bad secrets, you are too **small**.
If someone asks you to keep one,
 tell them, "NO, NOT AT **ALL**!"

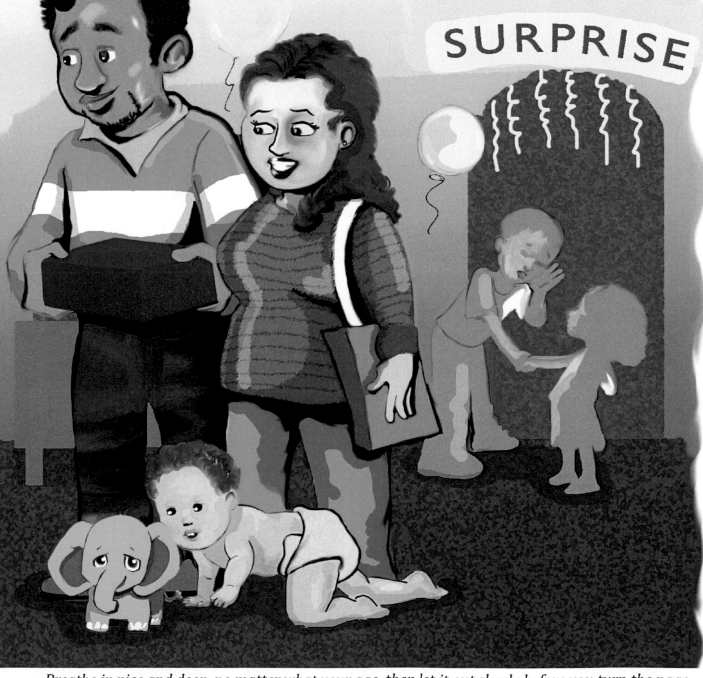

Breathe in nice and deep, no matter what your age, then let it out slowly before you turn the page.

Make sure to say it LOUD,
pretend you are 10 feet **tall**!
Then you do not have to feel
too young or too **small**.

If someone touches your body
or touches your private **parts**,
do not keep that a secret,
SCREAM with all your **HEART** ...

NOOOOOO
OOOOOOO
OOOOO
OOOO
OOOO
OOOO

Breathe in and breathe out nice and slow, breathe in really deeply, then let it go.

You are starting to see
that YOU are the **POWER**!
You glow brighter
and smarter
every day,
every **hour**.

You know that what's
below your *Tummy-Tum*
is not to **share**.
You need to know
so you can be **aware**.

Breathe in nice and deep, no matter what your age, then let it out slowly before you turn the page.

Tell everyone what you now **know**,
wherever you live, wherever you **go.**
Say, "I AM THE POWER, so remember my **name** ...
I DO NOT PLAY the-below-my-*Tummy-Tum*-touching-
game."

Li'l Lotus

Li'l Neshi

You can color **Li'l Lotus** and **Li'l Neshi**.
The many different colors are your **energy**: red, orange, yellow green, blue, indigo and violet.

Inside and outside the lines are fine.

Just create with the **greatness** you are.

Michelle R. Britto — Author

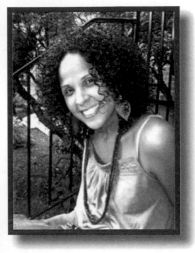

Michelle is a Licensed Social Worker, with a Bachelor's Degree in Psychology; a Masters Degree in Social Work; a Degree in Occupational Studies (the Body functions); and has a License in Massage Therapy. In her heart, she has always desired to be of service to humanity — especially working with children and adolescents. This has led her to work in areas such as Preventive Services, Foster-Care, utilizing alternative methods in Special Education, and her current position in the NYC Department of Education. She has worked privately with both adults and children, and in healing centers throughout New York City.

Her experience in adolescent and pediatric psychiatric facilities is what led her to explore a deeper understanding of the whole child. This allowed her to utilize the concept of how the interconnectedness of mind, body and spirit are beneficial when working with children. Michelle's degree in Occupational Studies (Massage Therapy) came as a result of the many stories of trauma and abuse that she heard as a counselor. Trauma which eventually manifested into physical ailments.

Michelle is a mother of 5 children who all came into her life as unique gifts. She is originally from Brooklyn and now resides in Queens. This is her first book.

Visit her on the web at: http://www.inlightenmebooks.com/

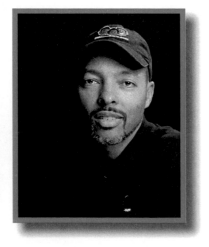

Photo Credit Hollis King

Jerry Craft — Artist

Jerry is the creator of "The Offenders: Saving The World While Serving Detention," a middle grade novel about bullying. He is also the creator of Mama's Boyz, an award-winning comic strip that has been distributed by King Features Syndicate to almost 900 publications since 1995; making him one of the few syndicated African-American cartoonists in the country. He has illustrated and / or written almost two dozen children's books and games and has won five African American Literary Awards. His work has appeared in national publications such as Essence Magazine, Ebony, and two Chicken Soup for the African American Soul books.

For more information, email him at jerrycraft@aol.com or visit him on the web at www.jerrycraft.net

Made in the USA
San Bernardino, CA
09 September 2018